Pulmonary Hypertension

A Beginner's Quick Start Guide to Managing the Condition Through Diet, With Sample Recipes and a 7-Day Meal Plan

copyright © 2022 Patrick Marshwell

All rights reserved No part of this book may be reproduced, or stored in a retrieval system, or transmitted in any form or by any means, electronic, mechanical, photocopying, recording, or otherwise, without express written permission of the publisher.

Disclaimer

By reading this disclaimer, you are accepting the terms of the disclaimer in full. If you disagree with this disclaimer, please do not read the guide.

All of the content within this guide is provided for informational and educational purposes only, and should not be accepted as independent medical or other professional advice. The author is not a doctor, physician, nurse, mental health provider, or registered nutritionist/dietician. Therefore, using and reading this guide does not establish any form of a physician-patient relationship.

Always consult with a physician or another qualified health provider with any issues or questions you might have regarding any sort of medical condition. Do not ever disregard any qualified professional medical advice or delay seeking that advice because of anything you have read in this guide. The information in this guide is not intended to be any sort of medical advice and should not be used in lieu of any medical advice by a licensed and qualified medical professional.

The information in this guide has been compiled from a variety of known sources. However, the author cannot attest to or guarantee the accuracy of each source and thus should not be held liable for any errors or omissions.

You acknowledge that the publisher of this guide will not be held liable for any loss or damage of any kind incurred as a result of this guide or the reliance on any information provided within this guide. You acknowledge and agree that you assume all risk and responsibility for any action you undertake in response to the information in this guide.

Using this guide does not guarantee any particular result (e.g., weight loss or a cure). By reading this guide, you acknowledge that there are no guarantees to any specific outcome or results you can expect.

All product names, diet plans, or names used in this guide are for identification purposes only and are the property of their respective owners. The use of these names does not imply endorsement. All other trademarks cited herein are the property of their respective owners.

Where applicable, this guide is not intended to be a substitute for the original work of this diet plan and is, at most, a supplement to the original work for this diet plan and never a direct substitute. This guide is a personal expression of the facts of that diet plan.

Where applicable, persons shown in the cover images are stock photography models and the publisher has obtained the rights to use the images through license agreements with third-party stock image companies.

Table of Contents

Introduction	8
All About Pulmonary Hypertension	10
Symptoms of pulmonary hypertension	10
What causes pulmonary hypertension?	11
Diagnosing Pulmonary Hypertension	15
Medical Treatments	17
Managing Pulmonary Hypertension	21
Pulmonary Hypertension Diet	23
Foods to Eat	24
Foods to Avoid	26
7-Day Meal Plan	28
Sample Recipes	30
Cod Burger	31
Shrimp and Egg Fried Rice	33
Trout Scrambler	35
Low FODMAP Blueberry Smoothie	37
Tomatoless Pizza	38
Vegetable and Tofu Chili Sauté	40
Stir-Fried Cabbage and Apples	42
Taste of Mediterranean	43
Hickory Tempeh and Broccoli Roast Bowl	45
Avocado Chicken Lemon Salad	47
Cobb and Egg Salad	50
Tofu Chow Mein	51

    Pad Thai   53
    Minestrone Soup   55
    Salmon Soup   57

Conclusion   **58**

Frequently Asked Questions about Pulmonary Hypertension 59
    Key Takeaways   61

References and Helpful Links   **63**

Introduction

Pulmonary hypertension is a condition in which the blood pressure in the arteries of your lungs (pulmonary arteries) is too high. This can make it hard for your heart to pump blood through your lungs and may eventually lead to heart failure.

Pulmonary hypertension is a progressive, debilitating lung disorder that can significantly reduce the quality of life and lead to early death. There is currently no cure for pulmonary hypertension, but with proper treatment and management, patients can enjoy a good quality of life.

Pulmonary hypertension is caused by a variety of factors, including genetics, underlying lung disease, and exposure to certain toxins. The condition can also be caused by heart conditions, such as left-sided heart failure or chronic thromboembolic disease.

A variety of medications are used to treat pulmonary hypertension, including vasodilators, anticoagulants, and diuretics. In addition to medication, patients with pulmonary hypertension may need to make lifestyle changes, such as quitting smoking, eating a healthy diet, and exercising regularly.

Pulmonary hypertension can be a difficult condition to manage, but there are a few things you can do to help keep your symptoms under control.

In this beginner's quick start guide, we will go into an in-depth discussion about:

- Pulmonary hypertension symptoms
- What causes pulmonary hypertension
- How pulmonary hypertension is diagnosed
- Medical treatments for pulmonary hypertension
- Proper diet for those with pulmonary hypertension
- Natural methods for managing pulmonary hypertension

So, read on to find out more about this condition.

All About Pulmonary Hypertension

Pulmonary hypertension can cause a variety of symptoms, including shortness of breath, fatigue, chest pain, and dizziness. These symptoms may worsen over time and can eventually lead to heart failure.

Symptoms of pulmonary hypertension

Shortness of breath

Shortness of breath, also called dyspnea, is the most common symptom of pulmonary hypertension. It can occur even when you are at rest. The feeling of being short of breath may worsen with activity or when lying down flat.

Fatigue

Fatigue is a common symptom of pulmonary hypertension, and can be caused by the extra effort your heart has to put forth to pump blood through your lungs.

Chest pain

Chest pain caused by pulmonary hypertension is often the result of the strain on your heart from having to pump blood against higher-than-normal pressures in your pulmonary arteries. The pain may be aggravated by physical activity or by breathing cold air. If you experience chest pain, it is important to see your doctor so that the cause can be properly diagnosed and treated.

Dizziness

One symptom of pulmonary hypertension is dizziness. Dizziness can be caused by low levels of oxygen in your blood. When your blood oxygen levels are low, your brain doesn't get enough oxygen. This can cause you to feel dizzy. If you have pulmonary hypertension and you're feeling dizzy, it's important to see your doctor.

What causes pulmonary hypertension?

Pulmonary hypertension is a condition in which the blood pressure inside the lungs becomes abnormally high. This causes the heart to work harder than normal to pump blood through the lungs, and over time can lead to heart failure.

Pulmonary hypertension has a variety of possible causes, including heart disease, genetics, underlying lung disease, blood disorders, and exposure to certain toxins.

Heart disease

While the exact cause of pulmonary hypertension is unknown, several factors can contribute to the condition.

Some types of heart disease can lead to pulmonary hypertension, for example, left-sided heart failure. When the left side of the heart is not able to pump efficiently, it can cause a back-up of blood in the lungs. This increased pressure can eventually damage the arterial walls, leading to Pulmonary Hypertension.

Patients who have had a heart attack or congestive heart failure are also at risk of developing this condition.

Genetics

Patients with pulmonary hypertension often ask what caused their condition. Unfortunately, in many cases the cause is unknown. However, some risk factors may contribute to the development of pulmonary hypertension, including genetics. Pulmonary hypertension can be hereditary and may run in families. If you have a family member with the condition, you may be at increased risk for developing it yourself.

Underlying lung disease

Pulmonary hypertension is a condition in which the blood pressure in the arteries of the lungs is elevated. This can lead to heart failure and death.

Pulmonary hypertension is often caused by underlying lung disease, such as emphysema or chronic bronchitis. These diseases damage the lungs and make it difficult for them to exchange oxygen and carbon dioxide. As a result, the heart has to work harder to pump oxygen-rich blood through the lungs.

Over time, this can damage the heart muscle and lead to pulmonary hypertension. Treatment for pulmonary hypertension often involves treating the underlying lung disease. In some cases, medication may also be prescribed to help lower blood pressure in the lungs.

Blood disorders

Some blood disorders, such as polycythemia vera (a condition in which the bone marrow produces too many red blood cells). Polycythemia vera is a condition in which the bone marrow produces too many red blood cells. This can cause pulmonary hypertension.

In polycythemia vera, the excess red blood cells can cause the blood to be thicker than normal, making it harder for the heart to pump and leading to higher blood pressure in the arteries of the lungs.

Treatment for polycythemia vera often includes taking medication to reduce the number of red blood cells in the body and phlebotomy (a procedure in which blood is removed from the body) to reduce the thickness of the blood. In some cases, a bone marrow transplant may be necessary.

Exposure to certain toxins

While pulmonary hypertension can be caused by several factors, exposure to certain toxins is one of the most common causes. These toxins can damage the lung tissue and cause the arteries to constrict, leading to an increase in blood pressure.

In some cases, the exposure may be due to occupational exposure to chemicals or other toxins. However, it can also occur as a result of smoking or inhaling secondhand smoke. If you have been exposed to many toxins, it is important to seek medical attention as soon as possible to avoid further damage to your lungs.

Diagnosing Pulmonary Hypertension

When a person experiences symptoms that may be associated with pulmonary hypertension, such as shortness of breath or chest pain, the condition is often first suspected.

Physical examination

To confirm the diagnosis, a physical examination and medical history will be conducted. During the physical examination, your doctor will listen to your heart and lungs with a stethoscope. They will also check for signs of an enlarged heart, fluid retention, and abnormal blood vessels in your lungs.

Your medical history will be reviewed to look for risk factors, such as smoking or exposure to certain chemicals. In some cases, additional testing may be needed to rule out other conditions that can cause similar symptoms.

When pulmonary hypertension is suspected, your doctor will likely order a series of tests to confirm the diagnosis.

Chest X-Ray

A chest X-ray is a painless, non-invasive test that uses low-dose radiation to produce images of the chest. A chest X-ray can often reveal changes in the heart and lungs that are associated with pulmonary hypertension. These changes may include an enlarged heart, an enlarged right ventricle, or an abnormal pulmonary artery. An echocardiogram, which is an ultrasound of the heart, can be used to measure the pressure in the heart and assess how well the heart is functioning.

Pulmonary function test

A pulmonary function test is a type of diagnostic test that measures how well the lungs are functioning. It can help diagnose pulmonary hypertension by measuring how well the lungs can move air in and out. The test can also help to determine if there is any obstruction in the airways. In some cases, the test may also be used to monitor the progress of pulmonary hypertension.

Echocardiogram (echo)

An echocardiogram, also called an echo, is a type of ultrasound of the heart. It uses sound waves to create images of the heart chambers and valves. An echo can often reveal changes in the heart that are associated with pulmonary hypertension, such as an enlarged right ventricle or an abnormal pulmonary artery.

Cardiac catheterization

Cardiac catheterization is a test that uses a long, thin tube (catheter) to measure the pressure in the heart and lungs. The catheter is inserted through an artery in the groin and threaded through the blood vessels to the heart. Once in place, the catheter can be used to measure the pressure in the heart and lungs.

By evaluating all of this information, your doctor can develop a treatment plan that is tailored to your specific needs.

Medical Treatments

Treatment of Pulmonary Hypertension often includes medications such as oxygen therapy, diuretics, blood thinners, calcium channel blockers, and vasodilators. In some cases, a heart-lung transplant may be needed.

Oxygen therapy

Oxygen therapy is often used to treat Pulmonary hypertension. It involves breathing pure oxygen through a mask or nasal cannula. Oxygen helps to reduce the workload of the heart and can also help to relieve symptoms such as shortness of breath and fatigue. In some cases, oxygen therapy may be used continuously, while in others it may only be used when symptoms are present. If oxygen therapy is ineffective or not well tolerated, other treatment options may be considered, such as diuretics, vasodilators, and pulmonary thromboendarterectomy.

Diuretics

Diuretics are drugs that help to reduce fluid retention by increasing urine production. This can help to improve lung function and reduce the strain on the heart. In addition, diuretics may also be used to help control blood pressure and reduce the risk of complications from pulmonary hypertension. While they are not a cure, diuretics can help improve symptoms and quality of life for those living with this condition.

Blood thinners

In the early stages of pulmonary hypertension, blood thinners may be prescribed to prevent blood clots from forming in the lungs. This can help to improve blood flow and reduce the risk of further damage to the lungs.

Calcium channel blockers

Calcium channel blockers are a type of medication that can be used in the treatment of pulmonary hypertension. These drugs work by relaxing the muscles in the walls of the blood vessels, making it easier for blood to flow through them.

In addition, to improve blood flow, calcium channel blockers can also help to reduce the pressure within the blood vessels. This can help to ease some of the symptoms of pulmonary hypertension, such as shortness of breath and chest pain.

Although calcium channel blockers can be an effective treatment for pulmonary hypertension, they are not suitable for everyone. Some people may experience side effects from these medications, such as dizziness or headache. Therefore, it is important to speak to a doctor before starting any new medication.

Vasodilators

Vasodilators are often used to treat pulmonary hypertension. This is because they work to widen the blood vessels, which in turn improves blood flow.

The most common vasodilators used to treat pulmonary hypertension include endothelin receptor antagonists, prostacyclin analogs, and phosphodiesterase type 5 inhibitors. These medications can be taken orally, intravenously, or via inhalation.

In some cases, a combination of these medications may be used to achieve the best possible results. It is important to note that while vasodilators can be effective in treating pulmonary hypertension, they do not cure the condition.

Additionally, side effects such as headache, dizziness, and nausea are common with these medications. As such, it is important to speak with a doctor before starting any treatment.

Heart-lung transplant

In some cases, a heart-lung transplant may be needed if the other treatments are not effective. However, this is a very risky surgery, and it is usually only considered a last resort.

With treatment, many people with Pulmonary Hypertension can live normal lives.

Managing Pulmonary Hypertension

Pulmonary hypertension can make even everyday activities difficult. Fatigue, shortness of breath, and chest pain are common symptoms that can make it hard to get through the day. While there is no cure for pulmonary hypertension, there are many natural methods that can help you manage the condition. Here are three of the most effective methods.

Eat a healthy diet.

Eating nutritious foods will help your body to function at its best and can reduce the symptoms of pulmonary hypertension. Make sure to include plenty of fruits, vegetables, whole grains, and lean protein in your diet.

Exercise regularly.

Getting regular exercise is important for everyone, but it's especially important for people with pulmonary hypertension. Exercise can help to improve your lung function and reduce the symptoms of pulmonary hypertension.

Quit smoking.

If you smoke, quitting is one of the best things you can do for your health. Smoking damages your lungs and can make the symptoms of pulmonary hypertension worse. If you need help quitting, talk to your doctor about quitting aids such as nicotine replacement therapy or prescription medications.

Many different medications can help treat pulmonary hypertension. If you're living with this condition, work with your doctor to find the best treatment plan for you. With the right care and lifestyle changes, it is possible to live a long and full life with pulmonary hypertension.

Pulmonary Hypertension Diet

Pulmonary hypertension is a condition in which the blood pressure in the arteries of your lungs is too high. This can make it hard for your heart to pump blood through your lungs, and can eventually lead to heart failure.

Many different factors can contribute to pulmonary hypertension, but one of the most important is diet. Eating a healthy diet rich in fruits, vegetables, and lean protein can help to lower the blood pressure in your lungs and prevent the progression of pulmonary hypertension.

On the other hand, foods that are high in sodium, fat, and sugar can contribute to higher blood pressure and should be avoided.

If you have pulmonary hypertension, it is important to talk to your doctor about the best diet for you. They may recommend a specific plan or list of foods to eat and avoid, depending on your situation. However, in general, following a healthy diet is one of the best things you can do for your pulmonary hypertension.

Foods to Eat

Fruits and vegetables

Fruits and vegetables are an important part of a healthy diet. They are high in antioxidants and nutrients that can help to lower blood pressure and improve lung function. Try to eat a variety of colors and types of fruits and vegetables every day. Fruits and vegetables come in many different colors, each with its own unique set of antioxidants and nutrients.

For example, blueberries are high in anthocyanins, which are known to protect against heart disease, while oranges are a good source of vitamin C, which can help to improve lung function. Eating a variety of colors and types of fruits and vegetables ensures that you get the most benefit from these nutritious foods.

Lean protein

Protein is one of the most essential nutrients for the human body, and it plays a vital role in the proper functioning of the heart and lungs. The heart is a muscle, and it needs protein to function properly. In addition, protein is essential for the production of red blood cells, which carry oxygen to the lungs. Without protein, the heart and lungs would not be able to function properly.

That's why it's so important to make sure you're getting enough protein in your diet. Choose lean proteins like:

- chicken
- fish
- tofu
- beans

Whole grains

Whole grains are an important source of nutrition, providing essential nutrients like fiber and minerals that can help to regulate blood pressure. Pulmonary hypertension is a condition in which the blood pressure in the lungs is increased, and can often lead to heart failure.

A healthy diet that includes whole grains can help to reduce the risk of pulmonary hypertension. Look for whole-grain bread, pasta, and cereals at your local grocery store. These products will typically have the word "whole" in the title, or will be marked as "100% whole grain." Choose these options instead of their refined counterparts to get the most benefit from your grains.

Healthy fats

Healthy fats like olive oil and avocados are essential for maintaining good health. Not only do they help to improve blood flow and reduce inflammation, but they also play a role in protecting the heart and preventing disease.

While all fats are essential for good health, the type of fat you eat is also important. saturated fats, which are found in animal products, can contribute to heart disease and other chronic conditions. On the other hand, unsaturated fats, which are found in plants, can help to improve health and prevent disease.

Foods to Avoid

Sodium

Most people are aware that too much sodium can be bad for their health, but many don't know exactly why this is the case. When you consume large amounts of salt, your body holds on to extra water to dilute the sodium. This can lead to fluid retention and increased blood volume, which in turn can put a strain on your blood vessels and heart, and raise your blood pressure.

That's why it's important to limit your intake of processed foods, fast food, and canned soups, which are often high in sodium.

Fat

Obesity is a condition in which an individual has excessive body fat. Obesity is a risk factor for numerous health conditions, including pulmonary hypertension. Pulmonary hypertension is a condition in which the blood pressure in the pulmonary arteries is elevated. This can lead to right heart failure and death.

A diet that is high in fat can contribute to obesity. Fat is a type of nutrient that provides energy and essential fatty acids. Fat is also necessary for the absorption of vitamins A, D, E, and K. However, too much fat can lead to weight gain and obesity.

When an individual consumes more calories than they burn, the excess calories are stored as body fat. Over time, this can result in obesity. A high-fat diet can therefore contribute to the development of pulmonary hypertension. Examples of high-fat foods are:

- high-fat meats
- fried foods, and;
- full-fat dairy products

Sugar

Foods that are high in sugar can cause spikes in blood sugar levels, which can be harmful to people with pulmonary hypertension. If you have pulmonary hypertension, you should avoid these:

- sugary drinks
- candy, and;
- pastries.

Red Meat

Eating a lot of red meat has been linked to an increased risk of developing pulmonary hypertension. Try to limit your intake of red meat, or choose leaner cuts.

Alcohol

Alcohol can interact with some medications used to treat pulmonary hypertension and can also contribute to high blood pressure. It is best to avoid alcohol if you have this condition.

Caffeine

Caffeine can cause spikes in blood pressure and should be avoided by people with pulmonary hypertension.

Pulmonary hypertension is a serious condition that can be life-threatening. It is important to talk to your doctor about the best way to manage your condition. Eating a healthy diet is one of the most important things you can do to help improve your pulmonary hypertension.

7-Day Meal Plan

A weekly meal plan is beneficial in helping you watch what you eat, and make sure you're meeting your daily nutrition needs. You can either follow or modify this meal plan according to your preference.

Meal	Breakfast	Lunch	Dinner
Day 1	Taste of Mediterranean	Salmon Soup	Tofu Chow Mein
Day 2	Stir-Fried Cabbage and	Avocado Chicken Lemon Salad	Hickory Tempeh and Broccoli Roast Bowl
Day 3	Low FODMAP Blueberry Smoothie	Shrimp and Egg Fried Rice	Vegetable and Tofu Chili Sauté
Day 4	Cobb and Egg Salad	Salmon Soup	Pad Thai
Day 5	Taste of Mediterranean	Cod Burger	Tomatoless Pizza
Day 6	Low FODMAP Blueberry Smoothie	Shrimp and Egg Fried Rice	Minestrone Soup
Day 7	Avocado Chicken Lemon Salad	Trout Scrambler	Pad Thai

Sample Recipes

Cod Burger

Instructions:

- 1/3 cup cracked wheat
- 1-1/2 lb. cod
- 1 tsp. lemon juice
- canola oil cooking spray
- 1-1/2 cups cooked white beans, dry or canned, no salt added, rinsed and drained
- 1/2 cup chopped parsley
- 1/2 tsp. salt
- freshly ground black pepper, to taste
- 2 tsp. olive oil

Instructions:

1. Place cracked wheat in a bowl. Cover with 1/3 cup of boiling water. Let sit until water is absorbed, about 10 minutes.
2. Preheat the oven to 375°F.
3. Place cod on a baking dish, and coat with lemon juice and vegetable oil cooking spray.
4. Cook until the fish starts to flake with the center still translucent, approximately 7 minutes.
5. Purée white beans in a blender or food processor.
6. Remove fish from the oven, let cool, and flake into a large bowl.

7. Add cracked wheat, beans, parsley, pepper, and salt. Hand mix everything.
8. Form into burger patties. This can make about four.
9. Over medium heat, coat a heavy-bottomed skillet with olive oil.
10. Fry burgers until each side is brown, about 4 minutes on one side.

Shrimp and Egg Fried Rice

Ingredients:

- 3/4 cup long-grain jasmine rice washed
- 1/2 cup water
- 1 cup chicken broth, no salt
- 4 oz. large shrimps
- 2 large eggs, beaten
- 2 cups sugar snap peas, trimmed and cut into two
- 1 cup shiitake mushrooms, caps only
- 1 cup carrots, diced into 1/4-inch bits
- 2 tbsp. low-sodium soy sauce
- 1 tbsp. garlic, minced
- 1 tbsp. fresh ginger, minced
- 1/4 tsp. red chili pepper, crushed
- 2 tbsp. vegetable oil
- 1/8 tsp. ground white pepper

Instructions:

1. Combine and boil the chicken broth and water in a small saucepan.
2. Add washed jasmine rice.
3. Reduce the heat to low.
4. Cover the saucepan with its lid.
5. Simmer until the rice has become tender, and the liquid has vaporized.
6. Remove from heat.

7. In a frying pan, heat the vegetable oil for half a minute.
8. Add minced garlic, minced ginger, and crushed red chili peppers.
9. Stir fry using a metal spatula for about 10 seconds, or until the mixture has become fragrant.
10. diced carrots and mushroom caps.
11. Stir fry for about 1 minute.
12. Add shrimp slices.
13. Stir fry for another minute.
14. Add sugar snap pear halves.
15. Stir fry for a minute, or until peas have turned bright green.
16. Remove from heat.
17. Add beaten eggs, cooked rice, soy sauce, and pepper.
18. While still off the heat, stir fry for about a minute or two, or until the shrimp are cooked through and the eggs have set.
19. Transfer into a bowl and serve while it is still hot.

Trout Scrambler

Ingredients:

- 1 small potato, cut into 8 wedges
- 1/2 tsp. extra-virgin olive oil
- freshly ground black pepper, to taste
- 1 cup spinach
- 1 egg, scrambled
- 3 oz. trout fillet
- dash of salt

Instructions:

1. Preheat the oven to 375°F.
2. Toss potatoes, 1/8 tsp. olive oil, and black pepper on a sheet tray.
3. Bake until the potatoes are tender, approximately 10 minutes.
4. Remove from the oven, toss in spinach, and set aside.
5. Heat 2 heavy-bottomed skillets over low heat.
6. In a small bowl, combine the egg and black pepper.
7. Put 1/8 tsp. olive oil in one pan, pour in the egg. Cook while stirring constantly until it reaches your desired doneness.
8. Place 1/8 tsp. olive oil in the second pan. Cook the fish until lightly browned for approximately 3 minutes.
9. Flip and cook until the fish are just beginning to flake but the center is still translucent, for about 2 minutes.

10. Serve the spinach and potato mixture with the scrambled egg and fish.
11. Just before eating, season the eggs and fish with a dash of salt.

Low FODMAP Blueberry Smoothie

Ingredients:

- 1 cup frozen blueberries
- 1 tbsp. almond butter
- 1/2 cup almond milk

Instructions:

1. Throw all the ingredients into a blender.
2. Blend on high until creamy and smooth.
3. Serve immediately. Top with blueberries if you want.

Tomatoless Pizza

Ingredients:

- 1-10 oz. can refrigerated pizza crust dough
- 1 tbsp. olive oil
- 1 cup cream cheese, light and softened
- 1 cup sour cream, light
- 1 onion, peeled and sliced
- 1 garlic clove, minced
- 5 fresh mushrooms, sliced
- 1 tsp. dried dill weed
- 3/4 cup baby spinach leaves
- 1/2 red bell pepper, seeds removed, sliced into strips

Instructions:

1. Preheat the oven to 375°F.
2. Place the dough on a greased baking sheet. Press and unroll firmly to cover the entire sheet.
3. In a bowl, mix the cream cheese, sour cream, and dill until everything is smooth.
4. Spread the mixture evenly on the crust.
5. In a skillet placed over medium heat, pour in the oil.
6. Stir in the onion, garlic, mushrooms, and red bell pepper.
7. Cook for about 4 minutes. The red bell pepper has to be crisp still but the onion has to be tender.
8. Add the baby spinach after cooking.

9. Spread this on top of the crust.
10. Bake the pizza in the oven for about 15 minutes. Make sure the crust edges are golden.
11. Upon serving, slice into squares and enjoy!

Vegetable and Tofu Chili Sauté

Ingredients:

- 1 onion, chopped
- 1 stalk, diced
- 1 carrot, diced
- 1/2 chili pepper, minced
- 2 garlic cloves, minced
- 1 green pepper, finely sliced
- 1 cup finely diced tofu
- 6 tsp. avocado oil
- 1 tbsp. brown sugar
- 1 tsp. ground cumin
- 2 cups red beans
- 1-1/2 cups of diced tomatoes
- 1 pinch salt
- 1 pinch ground pepper
- 1/3 cup grated cheddar cheese
- 4 tsp. fresh cilantro

Instructions:

1. Warm serving plates in the microwave to keep the salad warm.
2. Heat the avocado oil in a saucepan. Sauté garlic and onion for 2 minutes.
3. Toss in the vegetables. Cook for 4 minutes, stirring occasionally.

4. Pour brown sugar and toss in minced cumin and chili pepper. Cook for another minute.
5. Add in tofu and cook for 8-10 minutes.
6. Drain red and green beans and add to the saucepan. Stir well.
7. Toss in diced tomatoes and pour 1/8 cup of water, mix well. Cook for 10 minutes over low heat.
8. Add pepper and salt to taste. Pour the contents into the heated dishes.
9. Sprinkle cheddar and cilantro leaves when serving.

Stir-Fried Cabbage and Apples

Ingredients:

- 1 shallot, thinly sliced
- 1/2 apple, cut into cubes
- 1/4 savoy cabbage, sliced thinly into strips
- 3–4 radishes, sliced thinly
- 1/2–1 tsp. coconut oil
- salt, to taste

Instructions:

1. Pour some coconut oil into a wok.
2. Add shallot and cook until translucent.
3. Add the cabbage, radish, and apples to the wok.
4. Stir-fry for about 5 minutes. Don't overcook.
5. Add salt to taste.
6. Serve while warm.

Taste of Mediterranean

Ingredients:

- 1 cup uncooked couscous
- 1 1/4 cups water
- 1 (16-oz.) can artichoke hearts
- 1/2 cup kalamata olives
- 1 (12-oz.) jar roasted red pepper
- 1/2 cup feta cheese
- 1 cup cherry tomatoes
- 1/2 small onion
- 1/4 tsp. chopped oregano
- 1/4 tsp. chopped fresh mint
- 1/2 tsp. pepper flakes
- 4 tbsp. extra virgin olive oil
- lemon juice from a single lemon
- a piece of black pepper

Instructions:

1. Start by boiling water and adding the couscous. Mix well.
2. Turn off the stove after mixing.
3. Cover the mixture and cool for 6 minutes.
4. In a separate container, combine the rest of the ingredients.

5. Place the mixture in the fridge for 17 minutes.
6. Mix the mixture with the couscous.
7. Serve chilled.

Hickory Tempeh and Broccoli Roast Bowl

Ingredients:

- Hickory sauce, to taste
- 1 (8 oz) tempeh block

For the broccoli roast:

- 1 head broccoli, cut into florets
- 1 tsp. balsamic vinegar
- garlic powder, to taste
- black pepper, to taste
- salt, to taste

For the guacamole:

- 1/4 jalapeno pepper
- 2 tbsp. diced red onion
- 1 large avocado
- 1/4 cup diced tomatoes
- 1 tbsp. chopped cilantro
- brown rice, for serving
- 2 tsp. fresh lime juice
- black pepper, to taste
- red pepper flakes, to taste
- salt, to taste

Instructions:

1. In a small pot, submerge the tempeh in water, enough to cover the pot.
2. Bring the small pot to a boil for 5 minutes, and drain afterward.
3. On a cutting board, transfer the tempeh and slice into thick chunks.
4. Transfer tempeh chunks to a skillet, and cover it with hickory sauce. Allow the sauce to marinate for 15 minutes.
5. Once done, sear the tempeh chunks for 2 minutes per side; brush once more with hickory sauce.
6. To make the guacamole sauce, mix all the ingredients. Stir well to incorporate then adjust seasoning depending on your taste.

Broccoli Roast Instructions:

1. Preheat your oven to 475°F.
2. Line a baking sheet with aluminum foil.
3. Place the broccoli, and smear with balsamic vinegar, salt, black pepper, and garlic powder.
4. Roast for 20 minutes until broccoli is semi-charred.
5. Serve everything together while warm.

Avocado Chicken Lemon Salad

Ingredients:

- 2 organic chicken breasts, skinless
- curly kale, a bunch, ribs and stems removed
- 1 cup of cooked wheat berries
- 1 ripe avocado, sliced, drizzle it with lemon juice
- 1/2 cup pomegranate arils
- 1/2 cup pine nuts, toasted
- pink peppercorns
- pea shoots

For the rosemary oil marinade:

- 1/2 lemon, zest only
- 1 sprig of rosemary
- 2 tbsp. olive oil
- sea salt
- black pepper

For the lemon vinaigrette:

- 1 tsp. Dijon mustard
- 1-2 cloves of garlic, minced
- 2 anchovy fillets, minced
- 1 small lemon, juice only
- 2 tbsp. extra virgin olive oil
- 1/2 tsp. lemon zest
- sea salt

- black pepper

Instructions:

1. Prepare the chicken by washing and draining with a paper towel.
2. Slice through the chicken breasts for the marinade and cook well later.
3. Using a mortar, mix all the rosemary oil marinade ingredients until you get aromatic oil.
4. Gently rub the chicken with the rosemary oil and marinate for at least 15 minutes at room temperature or up to 8 hours in the refrigerator. Occasionally turn over the bag during the day.
5. Preheat the oven up to 375°F.
6. Heat cast-iron skillet over medium-high heat.
7. Add in chicken breasts. Cook until both sides are brown.
8. Move the skillet to the oven and cook for about 7-10 minutes.
9. Using a whisk, combine all the lemon vinaigrette ingredients in the bowl.
10. Put the kale and lemon vinaigrette in a large mixing bowl. Use your hands to mix for about a minute or two. Adjust seasoning according to your preference.
11. Move kale on a serving plate, topped with avocado slices.

12. Slice the chicken and place it on top of the salad. Top with peppercorns, pomegranate arils, toasted pine nuts, and wheat berries.
13. For garnishing, add pea shoots.
14. Enjoy by serving either warm or chilled, with the grilled lemon on the side.

Cobb and Egg Salad

Ingredients:

- 1 hard-boiled egg
- 3 oz. skinless, boneless chicken
- 1/4 cup cherry tomatoes
- 1 slice turkey bacon, crumbled
- feta cheese, crumbled
- bibb lettuce
- romaine lettuce
- lemon juice
- extra-virgin olive oil
- herbs of your choice

Instruction:

1. Make the salad dressing with lemon juice, extra-virgin olive oil, and herbs. Set aside.
2. Combine the solid ingredients in a large salad bowl.
3. Pour the dressing and toss to coat the salad.
4. Serve immediately.

Tofu Chow Mein

Ingredients:

- 1 16 oz. extra firm tofu, cut into 1/2" cubes
- 1 medium sweet red pepper, julienned
- 2 cups sliced fresh mushrooms
- 1/4 cup reduced-sodium soy sauce
- 3 tbsp. sesame oil, divided
- 3 green onions, thinly sliced
- 8 oz. whole wheat angel hair pasta, cook according to package instructions

Instructions:

1. Rinse cooked pasta with cold water and drain again.
2. Toss with 1 tbsp. oil.
3. Spread onto a baking sheet and let stand for about an hour.
4. Wrap tofu in a clean kitchen towel. Refrigerate until ready to cook.
5. Heat 1 tbsp. oil in a large skillet over medium heat. Add pasta.
6. Cook until the bottom is lightly browned. Remove from pan.
7. Heat the remaining oil over medium-high heat in the same skillet.
8. Stir-fry tofu, with pepper and mushrooms until the latter are tender.

9. Add pasta, followed by soy sauce.
10. Toss everything until evenly heated.
11. Upon serving, sprinkle pasta with green onions.

Pad Thai

Ingredients:

- 3 tbsp. vegetable oil
- 5 oz. pad Thai rice noodles
- 1 egg, large
- 2 tbsp. pressed tofu or bean curd, sliced into about half-inch cubes
- 1 cup bean sprouts
- 1 tbsp. sweet preserved radish (shredded), rinsed and chopped into one-inch pieces
- 1-1/2 tbsp. Thai fish sauce or nam pla
- 5 tbsp. tamarind water, or 2 tbsp. + 1 tsp. tamarind paste mixed with 2 tbsp. + 1 tsp. water
- 1-1/2 tbsp. simple syrup, a mixture of water and palm sugar
- 1/2 tsp. ground dried Thai chilis, divided
- 4 garlic chives, 2 cut into 1-inch pieces
- 2 lime wedges
- 2 tbsp. roasted and unsalted peanuts, crushed and divided
- Optional: 6 pcs. shrimp, peeled and deveined

Instructions:

1. Soak noodles in hot water until tender, for about 5-10 minutes. Cover it, but make sure they don't turn mushy.

2. Drain and set aside.
3. In a wok, heat vegetable oil over medium-high heat.
4. Add in the egg. Cook for about half a minute, stirring it until it barely sets.
5. Optional: Add in shrimp. Stir-fry for about 2-3 minutes, or until both are cooked through.
6. Put in tofu and radish, and stir-fry for another half minute.
7. Pour in the noodles and cook for a minute.
8. Add the sprouts, followed by the fish sauce, simple syrup, and tamarind water.
9. Stir-fry everything until the noodles have evenly absorbed the sauce, maybe about a minute.
10. Add in garlic chives, half of the ground chilis and peanuts. Mix well.
11. Upon serving, garnish with the leftover chilis and peanuts, along with the lime wedges.

Minestrone Soup

Ingredients:

- 3 large carrots, diced
- 2 large onions, chopped
- 2 cloves garlic, minced
- 2 cups celery, chopped
- 1 cup green beans, cut into half-inch pieces
- 1.5 cups kidney beans, dried
- 1 large bell pepper, diced
- 1 cup frozen peas
- 1 can tomatoes, diced
- 2 cups tomato sauce
- 2 tbsp. fresh basil or 1 tsp. dried basil
- 6 cups water

Instructions:

1. In a stock pot over medium heat, add the water, onions, carrots, and celery.
2. As the water starts to bubble, add in the green beans, bell pepper, peas, and tomatoes.
3. Let it bubble for around 30 minutes.
4. Add water if necessary. The soup should be thick, similar to a stew, but not too thick.
5. After half an hour, add the tomato sauce, beans, basil, and salt to taste.

6. Let it stew for 5-10 additional minutes at that point include the garlic. Let it stew for 5 additional minutes.
7. Serve while hot.

Salmon Soup

Ingredients:

- 1-3/4 cup coconut milk
- 2 tsp. dried thyme leaves
- 4 leeks, trimmed and sliced into crescents
- 6 cups seafood stock or chicken broth
- salt, for seasoning
- 3 cloves garlic, minced
- 1 lb. salmon, cut into bite-sized pieces
- 2 tbsp. avocado oil

Instructions:

1. Place avocado oil in a large saucepan or Dutch oven at low-medium heat. Add garlic and leeks.
2. Cook vegetables until slightly softened.
3. Pour in chicken or fish stock. Add in thyme and allow the mixture to simmer for approximately 15 minutes.
4. Season with salt to taste.
5. Add both coconut milk and salmon.
6. Bring the mixture up to a gentle simmer.
7. Cook until the fish is tender and opaque, then serve while hot.

Conclusion

Pulmonary hypertension is a condition in which the blood pressure in the arteries of your lungs is too high. This can make it hard for your heart to pump blood through your lungs, and can eventually lead to heart failure.

A healthy diet is one of the most important things you can do to help improve your pulmonary hypertension. Eating a variety of fruits, vegetables, and lean proteins can help to lower your blood pressure and improve your lung function. Avoiding foods that are high in sodium, fat, and sugar is also important.

If you have any questions about pulmonary hypertension or how to manage it, please talk to your doctor. With proper treatment, many people with pulmonary hypertension can live relatively normal lives.

Frequently Asked Questions about Pulmonary Hypertension

1. What is pulmonary hypertension?

Pulmonary hypertension is a condition in which the blood pressure in the arteries of your lungs is too high. This can make it hard for your heart to pump blood through your lungs, and can eventually lead to heart failure.

2. What causes pulmonary hypertension?

The exact cause of pulmonary hypertension is unknown, but it is thought to be caused by a combination of genetic and environmental factors.

3. How is pulmonary hypertension diagnosed?

Pulmonary hypertension is typically diagnosed using a combination of medical history, physical examination, and diagnostic tests.

4. What are the symptoms of pulmonary hypertension?

The most common symptom of pulmonary hypertension is shortness of breath. Other symptoms may include:

- fatigue
- dizziness
- chest pain

5. How is pulmonary hypertension treated?

There is no cure for pulmonary hypertension, but there are treatments that can help to improve symptoms and slow the progression of the disease. These treatments may include:

- medications
- oxygen therapy
- pulmonary rehabilitation, and;
- surgery.

6. What are the complications of pulmonary hypertension?

Pulmonary hypertension can lead to serious complications, such as heart failure and death.

7. Can pulmonary hypertension be prevented?

There is no known way to prevent pulmonary hypertension, but quitting smoking and avoiding exposure to secondhand smoke may help to reduce your risk.

8. What are the natural methods to manage pulmonary hypertension?

A healthy diet is one of the most important things you can do to help improve your pulmonary hypertension. Eating a variety of fruits, vegetables, and lean proteins can help to lower your blood pressure and improve your lung function. Avoiding foods that are high in sodium, fat, and sugar is also important. Talk to your doctor about the best diet for you.

9. What is the prognosis for people with pulmonary hypertension?

The prognosis for people with pulmonary hypertension depends on the severity of the disease. In general, the outlook is better for those who are diagnosed early and treated aggressively.

10. Where can I find more information about pulmonary hypertension?

The American Lung Association and the Pulmonary Hypertension Association are two good resources for more information about pulmonary hypertension.

Key Takeaways

- Pulmonary hypertension is a condition in which the blood pressure in the arteries of your lungs is too high. This can make it hard for your heart to pump blood through your lungs, and can eventually lead to heart failure.
- A healthy diet is one of the most important things you can do to help improve your pulmonary hypertension. Eating a variety of fruits, vegetables, and lean proteins

can help to lower your blood pressure and improve your lung function. Avoiding foods that are high in sodium, fat, and sugar is also important.
- There is no cure for pulmonary hypertension, but there are treatments that can help to improve symptoms and slow the progression of the disease. These treatments may include medications, oxygen therapy, pulmonary rehabilitation, and surgery.
- The outlook for people with pulmonary hypertension is better for those who are diagnosed early and treated aggressively.

References and Helpful Links

Eating healthy with pah: Diet & anti-inflammatory foods | cvs specialty. (n.d.). Cvsspecialty. Retrieved August 19, 2022, from https://www.cvsspecialty.com/resource-center/pulmonary-arterial-hypertension/eating-healthy-to-help-manage-your-pah.html.

Humbert, M., & Trembath, R. C. (2002). Genetics of pulmonary hypertension: From bench to bedside. European Respiratory Journal, 20(3), 741–749. https://doi.org/10.1183/09031936.02.02702002.

Mayo Foundation for Medical Education and Research. (2022, April 13). Pulmonary hypertension. Mayo Clinic. Retrieved August 19, 2022, from https://www.mayoclinic.org/diseases-conditions/pulmonary-hypertension/diagnosis-treatment/drc-20350702.

Pah-friendly foods: What to eat and avoid. (n.d.). Retrieved August 19, 2022, from https://www.pahinitiative.com/living-with-pah/pah-diet-exercise/pah-foods.

Pulmonary hypertension. (2017, October 23). Nhs.Uk. https://www.nhs.uk/conditions/pulmonary-hypertension/.

Pulmonary hypertension diet. (n.d.). Retrieved August 19, 2022, from https://pulmonaryhypertensionnews.com/pulmonary-hypertension-diet/.

Pulmonary arterial hypertension diet tips. (2014, April 9). Healthline. https://www.healthline.com/health/pulmonary-arterial-hypertension-diet-tips.

www.ingramcontent.com/pod-product-compliance
Lightning Source LLC
LaVergne TN
LVHW012037060526
838201LV00061B/4645